FUN FITNESS

LIVING A HEALTHY LIFESTYLE AND HAVING FUN

Dr. Fredina J. Weems

Gracednotes Ministries
405 Northridge St. NW
North Canton, OH 44720

Fun Fitness: Living a Healthy Lifestyle and Having Fun

Printed in the United States of America

Photography by Dave Cornelius

ISBN-13: 978-1719232999
ISBN-10: 1719232997

fredinaweems@sbcglobal.net

TABLE OF CONTENTS

Acknowledgments

1   Introduction   1

Fitness Barriers   3
Fitness Attitude   5
Family Unity   7
Mission Statement   8

2   Children's Fitness Program   9
Children/Teen Fitness Attitude   9
     Let's Get Motivated   10
     Exercise Preparation   11
     Children/Teen Fitness Mission   12
     National Standards for Fitness   13
     Components of Physical Fitness   14
     Children/Teen Fitness Class Pilot Group   15
     Children/Youth Fitness Fun Work-Out   19
      The Routines   19
      The Aerobic Drill   19
     The Resistance Drills   20
     Cool Down   21
     Words of Encouragement   21

3   Adult's Fitness Program General Population   23
     Adult Fitness   23
     Exercise Preparation   23
     Adult Fitness Mission   24
      Total Fitness Class Pilot Group   26
      Words of Encouragement   27
     Adult Fitness Goals   27
     The Routine   28
       Warm Up   28
       Aerobic Phase   29
       Work-outs   31
       Muscular Strength/Endurance   33
       Work-outs   33

Cool Down   39
Words of Encouragement   40

4   Senior Fitness Program   41
   Senior Fitness Goals   41
   Senior Pilot Group   42
   The Routine   43
      Warm Up   43
         Aerobic Phase   44
         Fun Senior Aerobic Program   45
Muscular Strength/Endurance   46
      Range of Motion and Flexibility   47
      Yoga breathing with Abs Work-Out   48
      Cool down   49
      Words of Encouragement   49

5   Special Population   51
   Accomplishments   51
   Multiple Sclerosis and Cerebral Palsy   51
      Exercise Preparation   52
   Fitness Goals   52
   Work-Outs   53
   Cool Down   55
   Words of Encouragement   55

6   Summary   56

Photo Illustrations   58

About the Author   66

ACKNOWLEDGMENTS

This book was written with guidance from God, words of wisdom from my mother, Estella Usher, who has gone on to be with the Lord, and the love of my father, Fred Usher. It took persistence, which my loving siblings, Pristella Usher, Rebecca Perry, and Herman Perry (my brother-in-law), made sure I maintained. I also want to thank my nephews, LeAnder and Ivoe Nicholson, who always believed in and supported my fitness journey.

I want to thank my husband, soul mate, and love of my life, Byron Weems, who supported me through the challenging times, sleepless nights, morning prayers and chats, and for his willingness to try out the various creative fitness ideas without a complaint.

I want to thank all of my work-out partners for their time, energy, and dedication to our daily exercise gatherings.

I want to thank my many friends, associates, and relatives for our brainstorming sessions, editing parties, and marketing skills.

I want to thank the Cleveland Clinic, St. Vincent Charity Hospital, and the St. Aldabert Summer Enrichment Program for allowing me the use of their facilities where I piloted and launched several successful fitness programs.

I want to thank my Fitness Trainer, Simpson Houston, CEO of Five Swords Martial Arts, for generously sharing his professional knowledge of Kenpo Martial Arts.

Again, I want to thank God for his mercy and grace, and for providing the opportunity for me to use this book to help others develop and maintain a fit lifestyle.

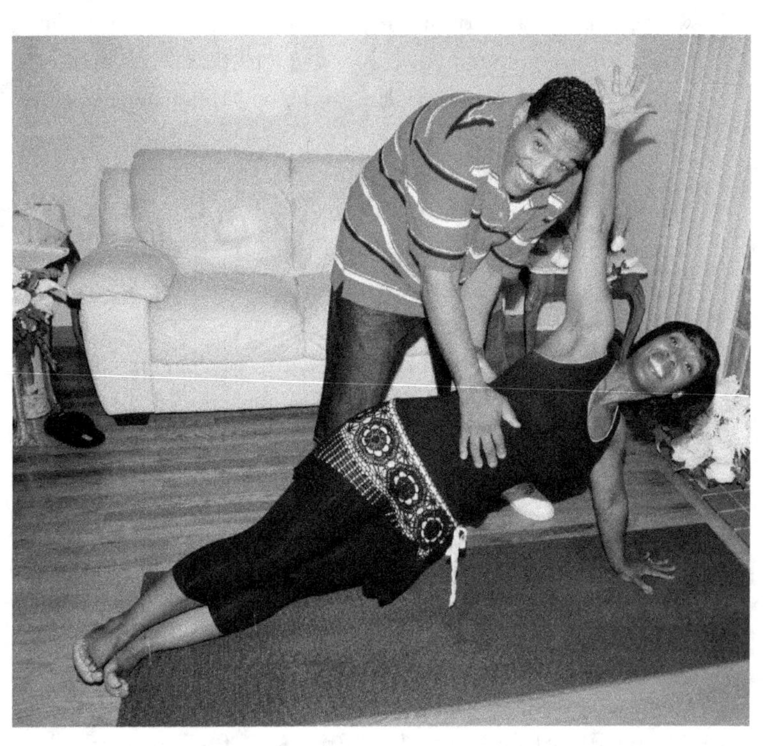

1

INTRODUCTION

Welcome

My passion in life, especially in the area of health and fitness, is to assist children, teenagers, adults, senior citizens, and the special needs population in living a long, productive, healthy, and fit lifestyle. Throughout my professional and personal fitness journey, I have encountered numerous people who have the desire to establish a lifestyle that includes physical activity, healthy eating habits, and positive self-image as its foundation. However, a lack of self-motivation, knowledge, and creative ideas can cause them to fail in this goal. This book will motivate, educate, and introduce my work-out partners (children, teenagers, adults, senior citizens, and the multiple sclerosis and cerebral palsy population) to ways they can implement and maintain a daily healthy lifestyle in a creative and fun environment.

We all want a lifestyle with minimum physical injury (knee sprain, back strain, hip re-location, shin splints, etc.), fewer health issues (diabetes, heart attack, stroke, high blood pressure, high cholesterol, etc.), and peace, unity, and harmony with family, peers, and co-workers. However, our daily journey is often filled with various stressful situations and unforeseen challenges. These obstacles require responses that produce peaceful outcomes, which occur only if our lifestyles include a positive physical and spiritual self-image. This fitness book will creatively encourage all work-out partners, in a fun and friendly environment, to enjoy life, accept their self-image, and exercise through daily challenges.

I assure my work-out partners that they will develop various fitness skills in a safe, educational, and enjoyable atmosphere. Having a fitness routine enhances consciousness of body composition and increases the benefit of sustaining fitness for people of all ages. Those with special needs will enjoy empowerment through the accomplishment of their individualized fitness programs while developing increased muscle endurance and strength.

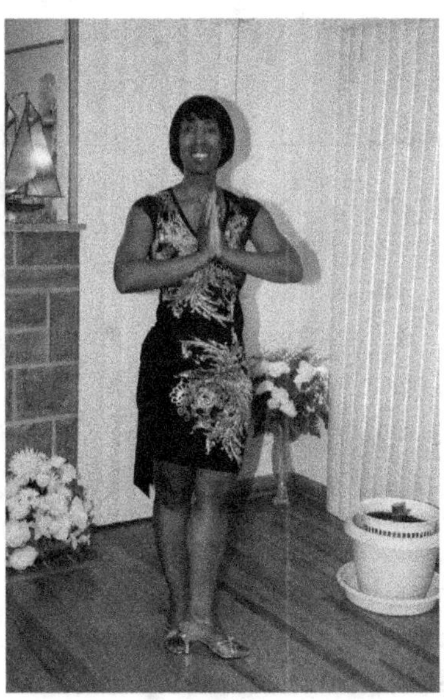

Fitness Barriers

Before establishing a permanent fitness program, we must recognize and eliminate barriers that block our fitness goals. Fitness barriers are obstacles that hinder our abilities to focus on and maintain a healthy physical lifestyle. Barriers can appear in various forms, both personal (internal) and environmental (external).

We can choose to have personal barriers. These barriers arise from how we see ourselves and how we decide to take care of ourselves. Selective eating of nutritious foods (such as vegetables, fruits, and whole grain) produces a high energy level, increases alertness, and positively affects personality. Consuming food high in starch and refined sugar (candies, pops, and chips) produces a low energy level, decreases alertness, and negatively affects personality. We all have weddings, birthdays and family reunions that provide fun family activities along with a variety of food choices. We should enjoy all foods (ex: desserts, vegetables, fruits, meats, and poultry) in moderation and within a healthy eating plan. If we know we are attending a wedding on Friday, our food intake the week before the event should focus on nutritious meals. This means no junk foods the week before the event. Eating dessert is reserved that week for the wedding event.

Next, achieving optimum health means acquiring a healthy internal self-image. The media often portrays physically fit women as sexy, slim, and desirable, while the sports articles illustrate men as body builders, with six packs abs and a sculpted chest. Both images are unrealistic goals for the U.S. female and male population.

God created us all uniquely, and we're fearfully and wonderfully made to cherish our individuality. A healthy appearance is more than just a Ken or Barbie doll image. It is the result of making healthy lifestyle choices.

External barriers can stunt our fitness journey. The opinions of peers and co-workers should be considered when they promote a positive or corrective influence that will assist us to achieve healthy fitness goals. The loss of a job or the start of new employment are circumstances which can be viewed as challenges that produce an attitude to motivate a person to engage in breathing meditations, aerobic classes and resistance training as preparation for job interviews or a new job orientation. Marriage or divorce are stressful times to be viewed as planned or unforeseen life changes, and can be supported through cardiovascular activities, toning classes, appropriate rest, and good eating habits to control cholesterol levels and maintain good blood pressure.

We can view our genetic family inheritance as gifts from God and as areas that we need to be realistically aware of as we adapt to various environmental changes. As an example, we can minimize our genetic risk of having a heart attack if we develop and maintain an on-going fitness plan. We all have fitness barriers that change our living conditions. Trying to maintain a health and fitness balance within a society that is constantly changing is why a fit lifestyle is a vital necessity. Refocusing our minds on images of successful fitness goals will eliminate the old self-image of failure. A successful fitness roadmap will mean seeing one's fitness dream become reality.

Fitness Attitude

A participant's attitude toward fitness and how they relate to lifestyle choices must be dealt with before individuals can accomplish their fitness goals. Self-image is important when relating to fitness expectations. A question to ask oneself is, "How do I envision myself physically?" Acceptance of one's current thought life and commitment to changes are necessities. This mental attitude allows for the refurbishing and redesigning of one's body frame. The question to ask is, "Am I willing to make the changes necessary to achieve my goals?" Meditating on success versus defeat leads to one's dream physique. Failure triumphs when an individual does not understand the relationship between mental awareness and self-discipline. Past failures have to be buried.

An individual's fitness goals should have a pace-setter rather than a past-setter mentality. Previous failures and deficiency of faith must be addressed. One's lifestyle is limited if an individual chooses not to acknowledge failed diets, weight gain/weight loss, or a slothful spirit. A daily mental attitude check-up is mandatory.

A key to reaching one's fitness goals is motivation. Daily living brings a variety of unforeseen circumstances. How people choose to respond to day-by-day trials affects their physical and mental attitude. The daily question to ask is, "What motivates me?" Motivation is a choice. Living an inspirational lifestyle means focusing on the following features: physical appearance, mental state, and health issues. Motivation must coincide with a willingness to change unhealthy behavior patterns. The motivating factors for developing/maintaining a good physical shape are health issues, career, instructors, loved ones and personal reasons.

Building a strong motivational plan will prevent participants from reverting back to past fitness failures. Speaking words of faith helps exercisers overcome past fitness tragedies. Opening our heart and mind to the awareness that we were created in God's image produces mental and physical rewards. Healthy living is an option when an individual realizes and accepts his/her identity and self-worth. Lifestyle responsibilities include mental, physical, and spiritual maintenance.

The mind must be programmed to see and expect to reach its daily fitness goals. We will operate only in a positive "thought" environment. A positive thought environment is one in which physical fitness goals are accomplished with determination, dedication, and continuous work-out.

The mind programmed for success must coordinate with punching in on a scheduled daily fitness clock. A good physical self-image will manifest as we cardio cross-train, sculpt and tone our muscles, as well as receive adequate rest. The mind and body are of one accord; remember, daily work-outs and faith are a team effort.

As discussed in the Fitness Attitude section, what we believe and tell ourselves daily will affect our physical out-put. Past fitness goals and life accomplishments were first possible as we perceived them, and then we achieved them. The mental preparation for achievement is guaranteed to start the fitness wheel in motion down the success road, pick up the physical activity steering wheel, and set the mind's cruise control button on automatic pilot for fitness victory.

Family Unity

All of our fitness information can be used as a chain of influence to assist our loved ones in developing or maintaining a lifestyle of fitness. Fitness teamwork within our families promotes an atmosphere of physical and mental encouragement. It allows us to transfer learned fitness information between generations in a loving and peaceful environment.

Family unity throughout our work-outs shapes the energy level, assists children's consciousness of self-awareness and self-respect, permits parents to proudly illustrate their fitness lifestyle, and allows grandparents to joyfully share their experience of aging with fitness. As I initiated and maintained my two nephews' daily fitness routine and spiritual growth, we enjoyed our family bond of physically working out together. Now Ivoe, who is in the military, and LeAnder, who is pursuing his dream of working in the movie industry, have a daily ritual of spending time with God and working out. Our family tradition is launching into the next generation.

Just as a chain of rivers from small to large connects and unifies into a powerful universal stream of continuous flow, family unity provides high energy levels, words of encouragement and love. Exercising together strengthens family bonds, promotes physical activity, and enhances healthy living in a non-competitive environment. Now that we know our family is our refuge, let us energetically moved forward to the Fitness Fun mission statement.

Mission Statement

By choice, we are active. Promoting exercise through fun activities will allow fellow partners to develop/maintain long-term healthy behavioral changes and stay physically fit throughout their life span. As a holistic fitness role model, I want to encourage youth and children, adults, seniors, and those in special populations to develop and maintain a fit lifestyle. am here to show all work-out partners how fitness can be fun, creative, challenging and beneficial to daily living. Their newfound fitness ritual will enhance their awareness of healthy body composition and the benefits of sustaining fitness. Special populations will be empowered by increasing their muscle endurance and strength, and by physical accomplishments through this unique, individualized, holistic fitness program. This fitness process prepares people for successful economic, social and productive living, as it occurred with my family. Also, this program was piloted successfully throughout Ohio. It's time to have fun with our children.

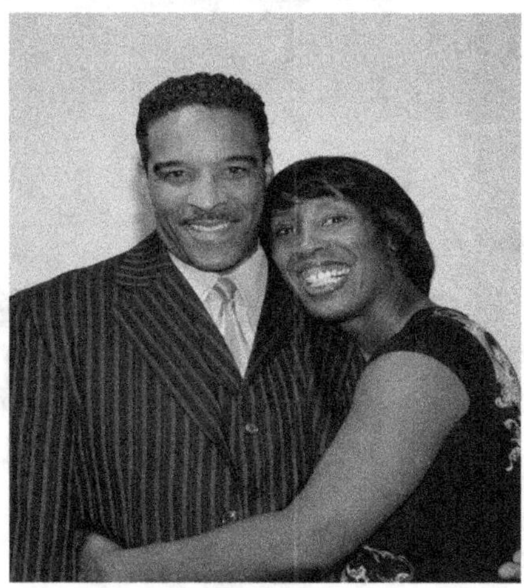

2

CHILDREN/YOUTH FITNESS PROGRAM GENERAL POPULATION

Children/Teen Fitness Attitude

Appearance is important. Society values appearance based on persons whose clothing sizes are from one to four. Self-acceptance for children and teenagers is based on the approval of family members and classmates, and often based on the example of entertainers. The transitional period from childhood to adolescence can either produce stress or peer pressure growth challenges, emotional challenges, or can provide self-acceptance of body type which was wonderfully created by God.

Destructive self-images are revealed as lean body frames, advertised by the media, are visually seen as the thin models stroll down the walkway. This can emotionally challenge teens to view themselves as overweight. Therefore, they develop eating disorders that are acceptable within society even though they are health endangerments. The acceptance of their body image by young people defeats the pressure to conform to society's unhealthy idea of body image.

Health and fitness goals include love and acceptance of one's self or one's identity, and a plan that adjusts and helps reach an optimal wellness level. The optimal wellness level includes the recognition of our family tree regarding health issues, our starting weight, and desirable and obtainable lifetime fitness goals.

Let's Get Motivated

While Lebron James credits his acrobatic performance on the basketball court to his daily commitment to exercise, Ali Michael, the teen fashion model, stated that her career suffered because of her eating disorders. The fashion and music industry often defines teen beauty and fitness by extreme dieting, glamour and buff physique. This type of look has caused and motivated teens to succumb to anorexia, bulimia, and diet pill addiction. Instead, teen music and fashion industries should try to influence and encourage a "healthy" physical appearance. This would eliminate or reduce health issues, promote self-acceptance, and encourage the building of a strong daily health and fitness plan.

Building structure for a solid fitness plan includes developing/maintaining our mental state as a place of peace, love, and contentment within the world of fashion and beauty. Remember, the world's influences, such as money, cars, rap artists, basketball stars, and the dream of becoming the next American Idol, cannot operate without the choice of acceptance.

As a fitness motivator, educator, and role model,

I encourage children and teens to choose the road that leads to a responsible lifestyle, including daily body, soul, and spiritual maintenance. Promoting fitness through fun activities allows development of long-term healthy behavioral changes and stay physically fit throughout their lifespan. This fitness process prepares children and teenagers for economic, social, and productive living while they pursue their dreams as a professional athlete, actor, or artist.

Exercise Preparation

The following conditions should be implemented before the child or teen's fitness journey begins:

1.   Medical Clearance: Health clearance from one's general physician should be obtained. This is required if he/she has health issues, and it is always good to check the child's health status (ex. diabetes, cholesterol, blood pressure, vision and hearing).

2.   Work-out Attire: Athletic shoes (gym shoes) are recommended to be worn during exercise classes. A white t-shirt (100% cotton) and comfortable shorts or sweat pants are appropriate work-out clothes for the adolescent to wear.

3.   Motivation: The most important component is to integrate creative fitness activities into a routine that will encourage and motivate him/her to stay active and alert. The routine should reinforce the benefits of physical movements, illustrate learning through fun, challenging activities, and promote the child's self-expression

and social interaction. The child/teen will gain under-standing of the various movement concepts, fitness principles, and exercise strategies to enhance his/her abilities to perform physical movements.

4. Encouragement: Parents, fitness educators, peers and family members should give words of encouragement to the young person before, during, and after fitness activities by verbally reminding them that each child is fearfully and wonderfully made. This will assist the participant to develop a long term healthy lifestyle.

Children/Teen Fitness Mission

This mission is to illustrate and explain the fitness guidelines in the following areas:

- Physical Fitness: This fitness definition includes muscle strength, cardiorespiratory endurance (aerobic) and flexibility.
- Strength: This helps them maintain healthy body weight and strengthen their musculoskeletal system, which reduces the risk of muscle injuries.
- Endurance/Aerobic: Fun, challenging cardio movements keep the children/teens healthy and energized.
- Flexibility: Stretching exercises improve their range of motion. This flexibility technique allows the joints to bend and reach with relaxed muscles.

Children and teens can benefit from physical activities. Those who continuously engage in an exercise program will:

- Enhance hand/eye coordination
- Develop and maintain motor skills
- Gain respect for self and others
- Foster teamwork among peers
- Become exposed to a wide variety of physical activity through a fun approach
- Decrease sedentary lifestyle
- Decrease the chances of becoming obese
- Develop and maintain muscle and bones
- Maintain lean body mass
- Decrease the risk factors for Type 2 diabetes
- Handle physical and emotional challenges calmly
- Lower blood pressure and cholesterol levels
- Sleep more soundly

National Standards for Fitness

The development and maintenance of good health requires physical movements. As the physical educator of this group I will use my expertise to educate and develop healthy students. The following fitness guidelines are recommended for children/teens:

1. Demonstrate their competency in motor skills and movement patterns during their physical activities sessions.
2. Gain mutual understanding of the physical movement concept, the movement principles, and the strategies and tactics that apply to the performance of an active life.
3. Note the importance of a daily exercise routine. An energetic lifestyle is the tool that enhances the students' physical activity for health, enjoyment, life challenges, self-expression, and social interaction.
4. Keep in mind the universal rule for achieving and maintaining their fitness level.
5. Take responsibility to respect self and others during gym time.

Components of Physical Fitness

The following health-related components of physical fitness should be the focal point of all our students' creative fitness drills:

1. Cardio Endurance: Use large muscle groups during physical activities for an extended period of time (this will depend upon each student's age, body rhythm, and his/her fitness level). Cardio activities should include short periods of energizing, vigorous on-going drills.

2. Muscular Strength: Use of muscle groups to exert maximum force against resistance (ex. push-ups and pull-ups).

3.   Muscular Endurance: Use of muscle group over an extended period of time against a sub-maximal resistance force (ex. repeated curl ups, ball toss, etc.).

4.   Flexibility: Movement of joints, without restrictions, through a full range of motion (ex. bend, stretch, twist, and turn). This fitness technique is used to make sure the students are properly stretching muscles, ligaments, and tendons to promote good body alignment.

5.   Body Composition: This is the ratio of body fat compared to lean body tissue. The focus point is how exercise and nutrition reduces excessive body fat.

Children/Teens Fitness Class Pilot Group

This creative, fun, and energetic physical activity format outline (summer camp 2007) was conducted at the St. Aldabert Summer Camp Program and piloted by Fredina J. Usher-Weems, with success (see table 1.1). Children under the supervision of parents, day care providers, or a fitness specialist can try this routine for at least six weeks and receive the following fitness benefits:

1.   Development/maintenance of lean body mass

2.   Decrease of the following health risk factors: diabetes Type 2, high blood pressure, high blood cholesterol level

3.   Decrease of chances of obesity and sedentary lifestyle

4.   Accomplishment of self-respect and social skills

Note: suggested timeframe can be altered based upon attention span of participants. With fitness assessment, record how many correct ones each child performs.

OUTLINE	AGES 5-7
Warm up: Timeframe 2-6 min.	Skip, hop (one foot, both feet, switch foot) jump, twist, lateral moves
Stretch: Timeframe: 1-2 min. (hold 4-6 sec.)	Neck, shoulders, biceps, triceps, back, chest, side, legs, toes
Main Event A: (Resistance) Timeframe: 8-10 min. (based on attention span	Fitness assessment: push-ups, jumping jacks, ab crunches. Drills between 1-2 min. Focus point: endurance and recovery
Main Event B: (Cardio) Timeframe: 25 min.	Aerobic moves: jog 1-2 min., freeze, skip 1-2 min., kickboxing, art kicks (3 sets of 10 each leg), jump rope (30 sec.) double Dutch jump rope (1 min.) Repeat routine
Cool Down and Clean up 2-5 min.	Repeat warm-up

Table 1 St. Aldabert Summer Fitness Camp Pilot by Fredina J. Usher-Weems (May 25-July 10, 2007)

OUTLINE	AGES 8-9
Warm up: Timeframe 2-6 min.	Knee lifts, silly, jacks, ski move, twist, front kicks (1-2 sets of 8 reps)
Stretch: Timeframe: 1-2 min. (hold stretches 4-6 sec.)	Neck, shoulders, biceps, triceps, back, chest, side, legs (upper, lower)
Main Event A: (Resistance) Timeframe: 8-10 min. (based on attention span	Fitness assessment: push-ups, jumping jacks, squats, ab crunches. Drills between 1-2 min. Focus point: alignments, posture and endurance
Main Event B: (Cardio) Timeframe: 25 min.	Aerobic moves: relay races (5-10 min.) kickball, ring games kickboxing, bike riding treadmill, jump rope softball, skating
Cool Down and Clean up 2-5 min.	Repeat warm-up

Table 2 St. Aldabert Summer Fitness Camp Pilot by Fredina J. Usher-Weems (May 25-July 10, 2007)

OUTLINE	AGES 10-17
Warm up: Timeframe 2-6 min.	March in place (50) Jump rope (25) Jumping jacks (25) Push-ups (6-10) Ab crunches (25)
Stretch: Timeframe: 1-2 min. (hold stretches 4-6 sec.)	Neck, deltoid, biceps, triceps, fore- arm, lat. pec ab/adductor (in- ner/outer thighs) quad, hamstrings, calves
Main Event A: (Resistance) Timeframe: 8-10 min. (based on attention span	Fitness Assessment: push-ups, squats, jumping jacks Main Focus: agility, recovery rate, stamina, endurance
Main Event B: (Cardio) Timeframe: 30 min.	Aerobic moves: Step drills (10-15 Minutes), Kickboxing, Cycling, Jazzercise, Hip/hop, swimming, jogging, volleyball, track, Cross trainer, Rock climbing, Soccer, Skateboarding
Cool Down and Clean up 2-5 min.	Repeat warm-up

Table 3 St. Aldabert Summer Fitness Camp Pilot by Fredina J. Usher-Weems (May 25-July 10, 2007)

Children/Youth Fitness Fun Work-Out

The Routines

The main point of having a routine is to keep it simple, challenging, exciting and most of all fun. The fitness drills should be between thirty seconds to two minutes in length. The cardio selection should maintain the children's attention span while exercising within maximum target heart rate. The chatter test can be used to verify intensity level. A moderate intensity level is preferred. The participant's intensity levels for the chatter test are as follows:

1. Light: Sing the lyrics to the entire work-out song.
2. Moderate: Cannot sing all the hip-hop lyrics but can talk comfortably (this is the desired heart rate zone).
3. Vigorous: Smiling but out of breath.

The Aerobic Drill

Feet to floor impact will determine the time duration of each exciting and stimulating aerobic drill. Jumping rope is considered high impact movements since both feet are off the ground. Therefore, the timeframe should not exceed 1 minute per session (example cardio drill should include jumping rope 4 times per minute). Marching is a low impact movement because it allows the participants to keep one foot on the floor at all times. This rhythm motor skill movement can be performed for at least 3 minutes and can be repeated for as long as it holds the child/youth's interest. Throughout the drills, make sure to keep the chatter test going, exercise within the fitness guidelines, and continuously engage and challenge his/her fitness level while he/she has fun. See table 1.1 for suggestive examples of cardiovascular work-outs.

The Resistance Drills

As the children are still within their muscle development stages, it is important to make sure the routine strengthens their musculoskeletal system while reducing the risk of muscle injuries. The amount of repetition and number of sets will depend upon each individual's range of motion and body alignment. Weight usage for children and youth should be minimum to light since they are still in the developing stage. If the youth is in athletic training, refer to his/her coach's guidelines. The weight recommendations are as follows:

1. Ages 5-7: their body weight, light resistance bands
2. Ages 8-9: their body weight, light resistance bands, 1-2 lb. dumb bell
3. Ages 10-12: their body weight, light to medium resistance bands, 1-5 lb. dumb bell
4. Ages 13-17: their body weight, light, medium, heavy resistance bands, 1-10 lb. dumb bell

Note: The key factor in teens' resistance training will vary according to their body weight, weight-lifting training, and weight tolerance level. Their weight tolerance level will depend on their muscle strength and endurance, range of motion, and body composition. The Fitness Assessment Test (table 1.1) used above as a resistance routine would be an excellent way to determine the teen's muscle strength and endurance abilities. To evaluate the youth's range of motion and flexibility, try various yoga and Pilate techniques (see illustration in the photo section).

Cool Down

After a work-out session, a cool down period is needed to restore body temperature to a calm and relaxing mode. Please do not skip this valid part of the work-out. Participants need to allow their muscles to relax and recover. This will reduce their risk of muscle injuries (see table 1 for cool down suggestions).

Words of Encouragement

Keep on working out and maintain a youthful outlook on life. Now that the children/teenagers are living and maintaining a fit lifestyle, it is time to assist or work-out with their adult family members. Remember we are a team that works out together (smile).

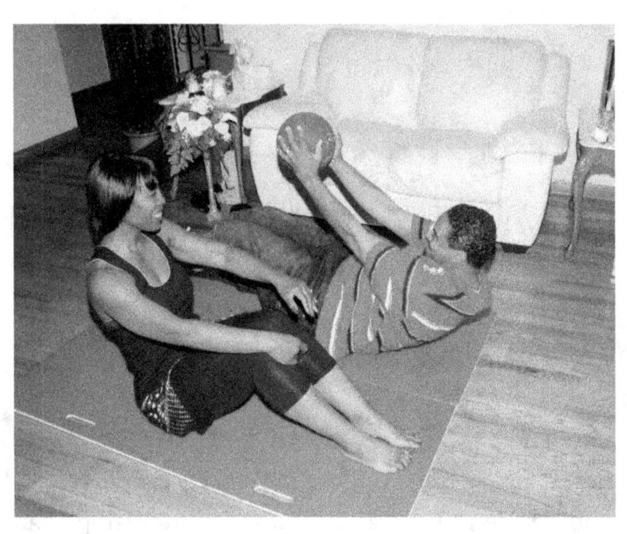

3

ADULT FITNESS PROGRAM (GENERAL POPULATION)

Adult Fitness

America offers adults all kinds of food choices, social events, career opportunities, entertainment places, wellness seminars, and fitness memberships, aily life challenges and poor choices have led to sedentary lifestyles, lack of fitness education, and have won adults positions on the obesity board.

Exercise Preparation

I suggest the following prerequisites before establishing one's fitness journey:

1.   Medical Clearance: Health clearance from one's general physician. This is required if you have the following health issues: diabetes, heart problems, high blood pressure, high cholesterol and/or live a sedentary lifestyle over the age of thirty-five.

2. Exercise Schedule: Plan work-outs according to one's schedule. The best time to work-out depends upon whether the person is a morning or night person. Exercise location should be based upon your preference, either a group setting (ex. fitness center, YMCA, health clubs) or individual environment (home).

3. Nutrition: How often and how many meals daily. A person must consider water intake. Water intake should be half your body weight per day if possible. Plan bathroom breaks.

4. Fitness Blockers: Know your fitness weaknesses and situations that would hinder your work-out time.

5. Attire: Athletic shoes are recommended (gym shoes) to be worn during exercise classes. A white T-shirt (100% cotton) and comfortable shorts or sweat pants are appropriate work-out clothes.

Adult Fitness Mission

The adult classes are intended to enhance a positive physical attitude through group cardiovascular work-outs. Encouraging words from the Holistic Fitness Facilitator will provide motivation and role modeling. The basis for this facilitator program is to assist the participants with functioning better when they believe someone genuinely cares. Through this work-out style, exercisers will reap the following benefits:

1. Improved self-esteem
2. Increased feeling of accomplishment and success

3.   Exposure to a wide variety of physical activities through interaction with instructor (combination of aerobic, anaerobic, core, Pilates, yoga, circuit drills, resistance training, breathing techniques, martial arts and flexibility)

4.   Decreased sedentary lifestyle

5.   Changed negative behaviors

Total Fitness Class Pilot Group

Fitness Goals	Partici-pants	# of Succes-sors	Comments
Self Confidence	20	19	Participants develop self-awareness and self-acceptance; enjoy their new looks and lifestyle
Health and fitness education and knowledge	20	20	Exposure to a wide variety of fitness activities gave them understanding of the necessity of healthy living
Sedentary lifestyle	20	20	Awareness of the following: active vs. inactive, energetic vs. lethargic
Behavior Changes	20	15	Awareness that negative habits/behaviors limited capacity to live healthy and led to health problems.

Table 4 The Total Fitness Group Fitness Accomplishment

The Total Fitness Class (winter schedule 2006), conducted at the Cleveland Clinic Fitness Center, piloted by Fredina J. Usher-Weems, was successful (see table 4).

Words of Encouragement

Whatever you set your mind to do, you can do it. If you think it, then you can start to accept it. Once you accept it, then you can believe it. Now that you believe it, you can envision your fit body. Finally, the vision of your fit body turns into reality. Now let us get started on your fitness journey.

Adult Fitness Goals

The majority of adults want to maintain a healthy lifestyle, yet most American lifestyles are sedentary. The purpose for Fun Fitness is to develop and maintain fun, injury free, energetic, productive, and active lifestyles. The following five fitness components are needed.

1.   Cardio-respiratory Endurance: Overall health and well-being include daily implementation of activities for enjoyment. Preferably, the duration should be thirty to sixty minutes, but three fifteen minutes sessions throughout the day are acceptable. Try this at least three to five times per week. The intensity level should be based on the person's physical/mental limitations. A person should always exercise within his/her target heart rate zone. This can be easily accomplished. If participants can enjoy their cardio time and hold a conversation breathing normally, they have exercised within their target heart rate zone.

2.   Muscular Strength: The fitness participants use their muscle groups to exert maximum force against a

resistance (ex. push-ups/triceps dip). Try two to three twenty-minute work-out sessions per week.

3.   Muscular Endurance: The exerciser uses muscle groups over an extended period of time against a sub-maximal resistance force (ex. repeated curl-ups). Try one thirty-minute session per week.

4.   Flexibility: The work-out partners move their joints, without restrictions, through a full range of motion (ex. bend, stretch, twist, and turn). This fitness technique is used to make sure the fitness participants properly stretch muscles, ligaments, and tendons, which promotes good posture. The timeframe for stretching is between eight and twelve minutes.

5.   Body Composition: This is the ratio of body fat compared to lean body tissue. The focus point is how exercise and nutrition can reduce excessive body fat.

The Routine

Even though the work-out will be creative, fun, and energizing, a regular format should be used: warm up, aerobic or resistance session, and cool down.

Warm Up

The warm up is an important segment of each individual exercise session. This time period is used to gradually warm your muscles up in preparation for more stimulating exercises. This period consist of five to ten minutes of exercise and stretches. Start with low impact movements such as marching in place, walking, and heel taps to get the blood circulating. The heart rate should not exceed the target heart rate zone (THR). The calculations for THR are as follows:

1. You will need to find your maximum heart rate (MHR)

a. First, subtract your age from 220 (ex. 220-35 = 185).

b. Next, multiply your MHR finding by 0.60 (185 x 0.60 = 111). This will represent the lower end of the THR zone.

c. Finally, multiply your MHR finding by 0.90 (185 x 0.90 = 166.5). (This will represent the upper end of the THR zone)

d. The numbers 111 and 166.5 represent your THR zone beats per minute; therefore, during your fun work-out, your heart should stay between these two numbers.

Next, stretch major muscle groups by holding the stretches for at least six to eight seconds. Major muscle groups that need stretching are your neck, chest, deltoids, back, hamstrings, quadriceps, and calves.

Aerobic Phase

Aerobic exercise includes using large muscle groups continuously in a rhythmic nature. The aerobic phase can be of one's choice. Remember, the more fun, the better the work-out and the greater the benefits. This session should be between thirty to sixty minutes, three to four times a week, and at a convenient time. The MHR is the calculation used for the high end number of your cardiovascular training zone. (See MHR calculation listed above in the adult's warm up session). An exception to this rule is if you are doing integral training or athletic training with a coach's supervision. See table 5 for various cardiovascular activities and calories burned.

Table 5 Selected Aerobic Activities

Activity	Calories burned/per hour
Running 10 mph	1, 280
Jogging 5.5 mph	740
Skiing (cross-country)	700
Running in place	650
Swimming (freestyle)	634
Step Aerobics	510
Aerobic Kickboxing	500-800
Walking 4 mph	440
Bicycling 6 mph	240
Yoga	198

Comments: Make sure the program is exciting by cross training. For example, for the first six weeks your cardio can alternate between power walking and an aerobics class (if your preference is walking and group classes). This time can be used to work on fitness beauty, health benefits, and body sculpting. The following are a couple of fun, challenging aerobic routines. Try them! As you progress, add and subtract to fit your needs and exercise taste buds.

Boot Camp Espresso Work-out

1. March in place 2-3 minutes
2. Stretch all major muscle groups (hold stretches for at least 8-10 seconds)
3. Push-ups (regular or modify): 10 reps
4. Hammer curl squats: 10 reps
5. Triceps dips: 10 reps
6. Jumping jacks: 25 reps
7. Basis squats: 10-20 reps
8. Diamond shape squats: 10-20 (take water breaks if needed)
9. Repeat above 2 more times
10. March in place 3 minutes
11. Stretch all major muscle groups (hold stretches 12 seconds or more).

Comments: Select a speed/endurance according to your body rhythm, goals, and endurance level. Have a fun, safe work-out.

Jump for Success Work-out

1. March in place   2-3 minutes
2. Stretch all major muscle groups (hold stretches for at least 8-10 seconds)
3. Jump rope 25-50 times (know your body)
4. March in place I minute
5. Jump rope 25-50 times
6. March in place 1 minute (water break if needed)
7. Jump rope 50-100 times (jump rope challenge)
8. March in place 1 minute

9.   Jump rope 100 or more times (grand slam) (water break if needed)

10.   March in place 2-3 minutes

11.   Stretch all major muscle groups (hold stretches for at least 12 seconds)

Comments: After three weeks, time this work-out to see how long it takes. The following week, try to beat last week's time. You can do it! Remember, victory is just a jump away. If you have a knee injury, check with your physician before trying this creative, fun work-out.

Fredina's Kickart Work-out

1.   Bob and weave 20 times

2.   Speed bag/squat 20 times

3.   March in place 3 times/ 1 knee lift 20 times

4.   Bob and weave 20 times

5.   Speed bag/squats 20 times

6.   March in place 3 times/1 knee lift 20 times

7.   Stretch all major muscle groups (hold stretches for at least 12 seconds)

8.   Water break

Drill One

1.   In fighter's stance, jab/reverse punch: 3 sets of 8 reps (right side)

2.   In fighter's stance, jab/reverse punch: 3 sets of 8 reps (left side)

3.   In fighter's stance, jab/ reverse punch right, jab/ reverse punch left: 3 sets of 8 reps

4.   In horse's stance, forward punches 8 reps, cross over punches: 8 reps, upper cuts 8 reps

Comment: Exhale as you punch, keep your abdominal muscles tight, have fun, and listen to your body.

5.   Four alternating forward punches, 4 upper cuts, 4 knee lifts right, 4 front kicks right

6.   Four alternating forward punches, 4 upper cuts, 4 knee lifts left, 4 front kicks left

7.   Four Jab/reverse punches (right) and 4 alternating front kicks (right/left)

8.   Four Jab/reverse punches (left) and 4 alternating front kicks (right/left)

9.   Four alternating forward punches, 4 upper cuts, 4 knee lifts right, 4 front kicks right

10. Four alternating forward punches, 4 upper cuts, 4 knee lifts left, 4 front kicks left

11. Four jab/reverse punches (right) and 4 alternating front kicks (right/left)

12. Four Jab/reverse punches (left) and 4 alternating front kicks (right/left)

13. Water break

Comment: Stretch all major muscle groups (hold stretches 10-12 seconds or more).

Muscular Strength/Endurance

Developing/maintaining a muscle strength and endurance program will decrease loss of bone density, which is a major health concern. A muscular strength and endurance combo package includes the following beneficial factors: muscle strength is needed to lift heavy objects; muscle endurance is used to assist one in sustaining repeated contractions throughout daily chores. Make this toning session exciting and challenging, not tedious and complicated. There are various strength-training work-outs. Feel free to select from the following choices:

1.   Total Body- This can be done three times a week with a rest day in-between each work-out session. This work-out includes working the upper and lower body within the twenty to thirty minute intense toning period.

2.   Upper body work-out- This can be done three times a week with a day of rest in-between training (ex. back fly, chest press, hammer curls).

3.   Lower body work-out- Use this session three times a week with a day rest in-between (ex. leg curls, leg extension, calve raises).

Your heart rate should not exceed the THR zone. Exercise routines should include a full range of motion. Don't hold your breath while lifting, as this will cause abdominal pressure. Suggested repetition and sets for resistance training are as follows: for weight loss, three to four sets of 15-20 reps with low weight, endurance training includes two to three sets of 8-12 reps with medium weight (consider your body alignment and fitness level), strength training routine includes one to three sets of 1-2 reps lifting heavy weights (depending on your body strength, alignment, and fitness level).

Strength Training Challenge

1.   Basic abdominal crunches: 10 reps

2.   Push-ups (floor or wall): 10 reps

3.   Triceps dips (kick back if you cannot do dips): 10 reps

4.   Ab crunches right: 10 reps

5.   Ab crunches left: 10 reps

6.   Basic squats (like you are sitting in a chair): 10 reps

7.   Calve raises: 10 reps

Ab Power

1. Basic crunches: 20 reps

2.   Bicycle crunches: 20 reps

3.   Ball crunches: 20 reps (on the ball)

4.   Reverse crunches: 20 reps

5.   Repeat the above 3 more times

Words of encouragement: You are doing a good job. Keep on crunching.

Work that Chest

Do you admire and appreciate a firm, toned, and sculpted healthy physical appearance? Do you need to relieve daily fatigue? Have you ever noticed that in the morning when you wake up, your chest is tight/stiff? One area that is most recognized for its great shape is the chest area. The chest area carries a lot of tension and stress. Below are a couple of chest stretch and strengthening exercises. They are good for morning, noon, or evening time work-out routines. Select a time that can conveniently fit into your schedule. Try to be consistent, determined, and enthusiastic.

Reminder: Remember to warm up for at least 5-10 minutes before you start a routine (Low-impact moves examples: marching in place, walking, bike, treadmill). Drink water before, during, and after your work-out. Always listen to your body. There is always tomorrow.

Chest Stretches

1. Clasped hands behind your back chest stretch
2. Place hands behind your back and clasp them together
3. Palms facing upwards
4. Pull your hands down and press your shoulder blades back and together
5. Make sure your chest is lifted up towards the ceiling
6. Hold your stretches 10-20 seconds
7. The stretch should be felt in your upper arms and chest
8. Try this for at least 3 times

Doorway Chest Stretch

1. Make sure the door is open
2. Stand directly in the middle of the doorway

3.   Place your hands on both sides of the doorway (shoulder height)

4.   Slowly step or lean forward to the most comfortable position (listen to your body)

5.   You should feel a comfortable stretch in the chest and front (anterior) shoulder muscle

6.   Hold this position for at least 10-20 seconds (listen to your body)

7.   Try this at least 3 times

Chest Work-out
Flat Bench Press

1.   You can do this on a bench or on a floor mat

2.   Equipment: barbell or dumbbells (weight preference is your choice)

3.   Lie flat on the bench/floor

4.   Knees are bent and feet firmly on the bench/floor

5.   Press back, shoulders, butt, and head, gently but firmly in the bench/floor

6.   Your arms should be placed straight up and shoulder width apart

7.   Inhale as you lower the weights

8.   As the bar/dumbbells reach your chest area, move the bar/dumbbells upwards

9.   Exhale as you push bar/dumbbells away from your chest

10.   Please do not bounce the weights off of your chest (This may cause massive chest/back injuries)

11. Try this for weight loss: 4 sets of 15-20 reps (light weights 1lb, 2 lb, 3 lb, 5 lb) or what you consider light weights

12. Try this for endurance: 3 sets of 8-10 reps (medium weight 5 lb, 7.5 lb, 8 lb) or what you consider medium weights

13. Try for strength/bulk: 3 sets of 4-6 reps (heavy weights 8 lb, 10 lb, 15 lb, 25 lb etc.) or what you consider heavy weights (Listen to your body.)

14. Stretch your chest (see the above chest stretches)

Seated Pec Fly

1. This can be done on a chair/bench
2. Sitting on a chair/bench
3. Chest lifted upwards towards the ceiling
4. Shoulders down/relaxed
5. Abdominal muscles tight
6. Spine in neutral alignment
7. Feet shoulder width apart
8. Hands holding weights of your choice shoulder width apart
9. Elbows should be in line with your shoulders
10. Brings elbows into your chest in line with your shoulders (bring them in close and in a comfortable position)
11. Inhale when you move the weights away from your chest
12. Exhale as you bring the weights into your chest

13. Try this for weight loss 4 sets of 15-20 reps (light weights 1lb, 2 lb, 3 lb, 5 lb) or what you consider light weights

14. Try this for endurance - 3 sets of 8-10 reps (medium weights 5 lb, 7.5 lb, 8 lb) or what you consider medium weights

15. Try this for strength/bulk - 3 sets of 4-6 reps (heavy weights 8 lb, 10 lb, 15 lb, 25 lb, etc.) or what you consider heavy weights (Listen to your body.)

Cool Down

It is important to return your body temperature to normal level. Cool down is a necessary phase of a work-out, which most people tend to skip. This relaxing time period reduces the level of adrenaline in the blood, allows the return of resting heart rate, and reduces the chances of dizziness and fainting spells.

Cool down format consists of five to ten minutes of low impact movements (ex. march in place, bike, and treadmill). Stretching all major muscle groups (holding stretches 10-20 seconds). This period allows participants to recover from their challenging work-out. Please end each session with two minutes of deep breathing for relaxation. Heart rate should be 90-120 beats per minute (the lower the better, depending on your fitness condition).

Words of Encouragement

Keep up the unity through family fitness and reap the harvest of family fun and healthy living. Now that we have children, youth, and adults aboard the lifetime fitness train, it is time to board the seniors.

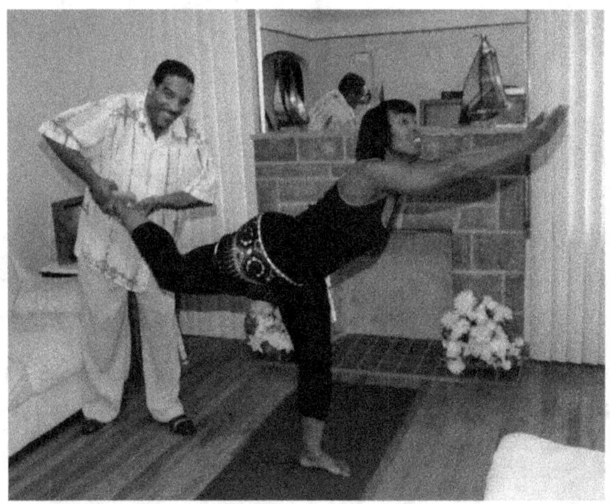

4

SENIOR FITNESS PROGRAM

Senior Fitness Goals

Life expectancy after retirement is a major concern of senior citizens. Living a long life requires a healthy lifestyle. Energizing work-out sessions will motivate and influence the older generation to develop more flexibility, range of motion, reduce their risk of injuries, and invoke a new beginning and healthy outlook on life. The following four fitness components are needed with the emphasis placed on the last three.

1. Cardiorespiratory Endurance: Daily implementation of low impact aerobic movements of your enjoyment. Preferably, the duration should be 15-45 minutes. Try this at least 3-4 times a week. The intensity level should be based on your physical and mental limitations. Exercise limits are within your THR zone. This will not be hard to do. If you can enjoy cardio time, and can hold conversation while breathing normally, you have exercised within your THR zone.

2. Muscular Strength: This relates to stabilizing your body weight while lifting objects. The senior uses

his/her muscle group to exert force against a resistance (ex. wall push-ups/chair lifts). Try this two to three times per week. Timeframe per session should be approximately twenty minutes.

3.   Muscular Endurance: Assists seniors with repetitive transitional movements. The exerciser uses muscle groups over an extended period of time against a sub-maximal resistance force (ex. gardening and repeated curl ups).

4.   Flexibility: Reduces the risk of hip, back, and foot injuries, which commonly occur among the elderly. The work-out partners move their joints, without restriction, through a full range of motion within their physical movement limitations (ex. bend, stretch, twist and turn). This promotes proper stretching for muscles, ligaments and tendons. Depending on your body temperature, stretches can be held five to thirty seconds. Stretches should be performed frequently.

5.   Body Composition: The ratio of body fat to lean body tissue. The focus of excess body fat is around the mid-section, chest and legs. Seniors are more susceptible to arthritis, heart attacks, hip dislocation, knee injuries and breathing spells.

Senior's Pilot Group

The senior citizens residing at Beachwood Towers, located in Cleveland, Ohio, served as the model group (50-75 participants). Their work-out seminars included Dyna-band resistance training. This technique led to self-confidence, increased muscle strength, flexibility and reduced hip fracture risk. Yoga was the stretch and flexibility format. As a result, the body alignment transformations were remarkable, which was important given the seniors' propensity for osteoporosis. Subjects reported reduced joint pain, which had been severe prior to their resistance training.

The Routine

The seniors' personalized work-out should be highly energetic and motivating. The work-out sequence includes warm up, aerobic, resistance training, and cool down.

Warm up

This preparation segment is very important. The warm up period is used to gradually condition the body for the aerobic phase. The time period is 5-10 minutes of exercises and stretches. This is used to get one's blood circulating and flowing throughout the body. Your heart rate should not exceed the target heart rate zone (ex. 220 minus your age at 60%, 220 minus your age at 75% [You can use the THR/MRH formula given in the General Adult Fitness Warm-up) Next, stretch all major muscle groups by holding the stretches for at least eight to thirty seconds. The major muscle groups that need stretching are your neck, chest, deltoids, back, hamstrings, quadriceps, and calves. (See suggested Cardio Work-out for warm up samples.)

Aerobic Phase

Aerobic exercise is one of the tools used to extend one's lifetime in an energizing way. The mature population should take into consideration body rhythm, flexibility, physical condition, and the body's range of motion. Cardio activity is performed for 15-45 minutes, 3-4 times a week, and at one's time preference. Try to remember to always adjust your work-out according to your body's limitation. Low impact cardio exercises are recommended for the fifty years or older age group. See Suggested Aerobic exercise. Remember the choice of exercise will depend upon your physical condition, and exercise expertise (ex: novice, experienced or seasonal exercise person).

Activity	Calories burned per 30 minutes
Walking 2 miles	220
Swimming (freestyle)	317
Bicycling 3 miles	120
Yoga	100
Pilates	100
Dance Class	75-100

Table 5 Selective Low Impact Aerobic Activities

Seniors, make your aerobic time fun, adventurous, and safe. Try various walking trails during the daytime. Watch your favorite program while biking. Yoga is the time for relaxing music and swim time is beach time. Do not forget to cross train. See below for suggested cross training cardio routine.

Fun Senior Aerobic Programs
15-30 minutes

Adventure Road Trip (2 days a week)

1. March in place 1-2 minutes
2. Stretch all major muscle groups (ex: hamstrings, quadriceps, back, and chest). Hold stretches 8-30 seconds.
3. Power walk 1-2 miles (take the scenic route. If on treadmill, let the sun shine in).
4. Dance in place, or around for 1-2 minutes.
5. Power walk 1 mile or treadmill (always remember to listen to your body).
6. Power walk 1 mile or treadmill (always remember to listen to your body).
7. Cool down 2-5 minutes, repeat warm up (above).

Swim Fun (2 days a week)

1. Jog/march in water 1-2 minutes.
2. Stretch all major muscle groups (ex. hamstrings, quadriceps, back, and chest). Hold stretches 8-30 seconds.
3. Breast stroke (2- 4 laps).
4. Jog/march in water 1 minute.
5. Back stroke (2 -4 laps).
6. Free style(4 laps.)
7. Jog/march in water 1-2 minutes.

8.   Fun Challenge- breaststroke 4 laps, back stroke 4 laps and free style 4 laps (you can adjust laps according to your fitness level).

9.   Cool down 2-5 minutes (repeat step 1 and 2 above).

The Bike Hike

1.   On bike warm up 1-2 minutes.

2.   Stretch all major muscle groups (ex. hamstrings, quadriceps, back and chest) Hold stretches 8-30 seconds.

3.   Bike trip phase one: steady pace 5 minutes.

4.   Bike trip phase two: speed 1 minute (adjust speed to increase on increments of 2).

5.   Bike trip phase three: steady go 4 minutes.

6.   Bike trip phase four: speed 1.5 minutes.

7.   Bike trip phase five: steady 3 minutes.

8.   Bike trip phase six: 2 minutes (know your body).

9.   Cool down repeat bike warm up.

Remember, this is fun and energizing. Enjoy the moment. Don't forget to drink your water.

Muscular Strength/Endurance

Between five and ten percent of muscle strength decreases and muscle tissue loss is noticeable in seniors who do not engage in strength training. Various health and fitness research studies have proven that physically inactive individuals, from the ages of twenty-five to sixty, lose 0.5% of lean muscle mass every year. Men will always lift more weight than women. Males have greater muscle mass than females. Muscle basis comparisons have proven that men and women are equally strong and experience similar rates of muscle strength and muscle endurance improvement.

To maintain strength and muscle mass, continuous resistance training is required. Every decade, after the age of twenty-five, women lose 5 lb/2.3 kilograms and men lose 7 lb/3.1 kilograms of muscle. Eventually, this will lead to strength deficiency and slower resting metabolic rate.

Range of Motion and Flexibility

In order to grow old gracefully, our physical bodies require exercises that permit us more flexibility and range of motion within our muscle-joint connection. We need to be able to bend without leg muscle tightness and reach for eye level objects without arm soreness. Yoga exercises have assisted seniors in maintaining physical posture and harmonizing their body, mind, and spirit through relaxed breathing practices. Try some of the following breathing and yoga moves: Yoga breathing with a hint of Abdominal Work-out

Quiet Breathe

1.   Lay flat on your mat in supine position (your back is gently rested against the mat).
2.   If desired, close your eyes.
3.   Relax your mind and body.

4. Inhale for four (4) counts (Hold your breath for 4 seconds).

5. Exhale slowly for four counts.

6. Repeat at least 5-8 times.

Yoga Abs
The Hundreds

1. Lie with your back on the floor.

2. Place your arms down by your sides.

3. Place your knees in the air directly above your hips.

4. Extend your calves parallel to the floor.

5. Exhale as you contract your abs to lift your shoulders.

6. Inhale and press your palms down rhythmically

7. Exhale 5 short quick breaths as you press your palms downward.

8. Repeat the sequence at least 10 times, if possible, which will total 100 breaths.

Comments: To challenge your endurance level, you can extend your legs while pointing your toes, and lift your head off the mat. Please make sure you do not feel any pressure in your neck. If you do, relax your head back onto the mat.

The Roll Up

1. Lie on your back and place your arms above your head.

2.   As your legs are being extended (straight with feet flexed), inhale.

3.   As you place your arms at chest level, exhale.

4.   Engage your abs, squeeze your inner thighs together, and lift your shoulders up towards the ceiling while bringing your ribs closer to your hips.

5.   As you roll up, allow the movement to come from your core versus momentum.

6.   As you roll up, keep your chin tucked to your chest.

7.   In a seated position, relax your shoulders, keep your abs tight, and inhale.

8.   Exhale as you bend forward, and keep your abs tight.

9.   Roll back to starting position, initiating this movement from your abdominal area.

10. Try focusing on feeling your vertebrae touch the floor.

11. Try these at least 3 times using slow and controlled movements.

Words of encouragement: You are doing a great job of maintaining healthy abs. Remember: slow and control movements with each step.

Cool Down

Now it is time to relax. The purpose for this session is to harmonize your mind, body, and spirit to its restored state. The cool down format will consist of low-impact cardio movements (ex: walking, biking), gently stretching all major muscle groups (ex: hamstrings, back, chest), and five minutes of breathing (try using the Quiet Breathe practice). Timeframe for this important session is between eight to twenty minutes.

Words of Encouragement

Now that we know staying fit has no age limitation, we can gracefully maintain a healthy lifestyle with fun and exciting aerobic and weight training routines. Our exercise family reunion consists of children, youth, parents, and grandparents. Next on our invitation list are our special needs family members (this population includes family members with Multiple Sclerosis, Cerebral Palsy, Diabetes, and Stroke).

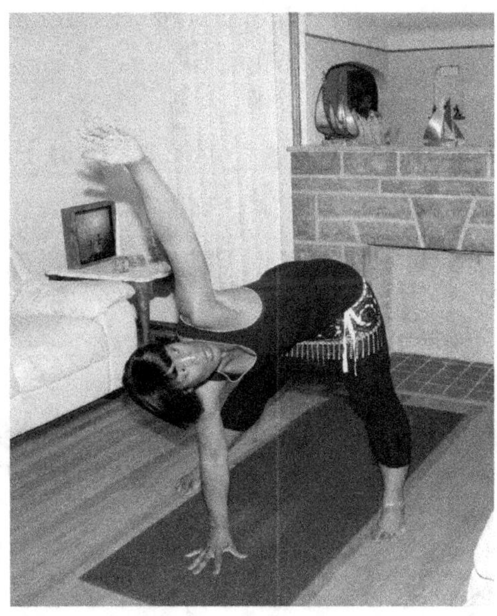

5

SPECIAL POPULATION

Accomplishments

Performing daily chores are considered accomplishments for our population with special medical conditions. Physical activities challenge and improve skill levels, muscle function balance, and coordination. Multiple Sclerosis and Cerebral Palsy exercisers can develop proper posture, increased joint range of motion, and decreased social isolation, thanks to physical activity.

Multiple Sclerosis and Cerebral Palsy Exercise Preparation

Before engaging in a daily fitness routine, check with your general physician and physical therapist to find out how your physical limitation and medication will affect your fitness lifestyle. Make a note of what climates will cause you to quickly fatigue. Aqua aerobic participants should avoid temperatures above 80 degrees. Outside fitness activities should be before 10:00 AM and after 4:00 PM. Please make sure you dress according to your body temperature, and take plenty of water breaks.

Suggested fitness guidelines are:

1.   Working out daily for 5 minutes with several 30 second sessions.

2.   Low-impact cardio sessions can include aqua cardio, aqua tone, and a stroll through the backyard or park.

3.   Light strength training sessions, which will allow you to use your own body weight, dumbbells (weight between 1-3 lb according to your physical therapists approval), tubes or bands (which weight equivalent is between 1-3 lb).

4.   Most important factor is that your work-out routines should progress gradually with success at every session.

5.   Check your intensity level by the chatter test

Note: Remember, You were created special and your work-out should be challenging but never fatiguing.

Fitness Goals

Moving from one destination to the next requires maintaining muscle mass, moving through your joint range of motion fluidity, and balancing your body weight while having good posture. With persistence and determination, our Multiple Sclerosis and Cerebral Palsy work-out partners can constantly improve their coordination, functional movements, and muscle endurance with their personalized fitness plan. See next pages for creative, fun, safe and effective work-outs.

Coordination Cruise

(Can use either your walker, dinner table, or a chair)

Circuit 1

1. Sit in the chair.
2. Take a deep breath and exhale. Relax; we are going to have fun.
3. Place your hands on the walker or dinner table (make sure your work-out partner is there to hold the walker or chair in place).
4. Slowly lean forward until your head comes close to the table or walker.
5. Breathe out (exhale) as your head comes close to the table or walker.
6. Slowly push away from the table or walker.
7. Breathe in (inhale) as you push away from the table or walker.
8. Great job.
9. Try this 4 more times.
10. WOW! It is time for a break (do you need some water?)

Circuit 2

1. Still sitting in the chair.
2. Close your eyes and breathe in (inhale), and breathe out (exhale).
3. Make sure your walker or dinner table is not in front of you.
4. Slowly see how high you can lift your right foot.

5.   Now see if you can bend your right knee.

6.   If you can or choose not to, hold your right leg up for between 5-10 seconds (you count from 1-10).

7.   Slowly lower your right leg down.

8.   Great job.

9.   Let us try this on the left side.

10.   Do you think you can lift them both? Let us try and see (smile).

11.   Nice job. Now, let us repeat this 1 more time.

Circuit 3 (Aerobic)

1.   Select a cardio (ex: Aqua, cycling, or a stroll).

2.   Make sure your work-out partner is with you having fun.

3.   Try this for 5 minutes daily.

4.   You can cross train (ex: day 1 aqua, day 2, cycling, day 3 stroll, etc.).

5.   Aqua day – try floating on the water (make sure you have your life jacket on).

6.   Stroll – walking around a tree or from one chair to the next.

7.   Cycling – slow and 4 intervals of 1 minute paddling.

8.   It is time to rest and look at the progress you made. You should be proud of the progress you have made.

9.   See you tomorrow. You can do it.

Hand Power

1. Sitting in your favorite chair.
2. Place a tennis ball in your right hand.
3. Slowly squeeze the ball for 2-6 seconds.
4. Relax your right hand muscle.
5. Try slowly squeezing the ball in your right hand again for 5-8 seconds.
6. Relax your right hand muscle.
7. At your own pace, place the ball in your left hand.
8. Slowly squeeze the ball for 2-6 seconds.
9. Relax your left hand muscle.
10. Try slowly squeezing the ball in your left hand again for 5-8 seconds.
11. Great job, let us cool down.

Cool Down

Gentle Breathing
1. Close your eyes.
2. Calm your mind.
3. Inhale for 2-5 counts.
4. Exhale slowly for 5 counts
5. Repeat for as many times that you feel necessary.

Words of Encouragement

Wow! What a great job. It is now time for us to celebrate your accomplishment within our family unity.

6

SUMMARY

Learning to love, respect, and appreciate ourselves is necessary for a successful healthy image. Our fitness journey requires uniformity with our spirit, soul, and body. Acceptance and approval from family, peers, and co-workers can be channeled through social group events, employment, or religious gatherings. From the time we are born until we die, we will interact with family. Our fitness journey should include remembrance of our loved ones sharing fitness words of wisdom and a visual photo of family exercising as a team.

Life is a road full of daily un-expected twists, curves and turns. As I reflect back over my family fitness journey, we have laughed together, cried together, and continued to exercise together. We have experienced the death of loved ones, marital problems, and health issues; however, our family exercise ritual continues.

As our children develop and maintain their perceptual motor skills, their adventurous and energetic personality contributes to our family fitness. The adolescent's concern of having a physically fit image motivates our families to have a consistent daily exercise plan. Parents' intentions are to maintain family unity and assist us through fun and challenging work-outs. Grandparents' love for their grandchildren encourages them to live long, productive lives. Finally, for our family members of the special population, their fitness goals include strength training to assist them in transporting their own body weight.

We can make the journey smooth by enjoying our family, by motivating one another and committing to assist each other in developing and maintaining healthy lifestyles through engaging in family creative Fun Fitness.

PHOTO ILLUSTRATIONS

Table Push-Up

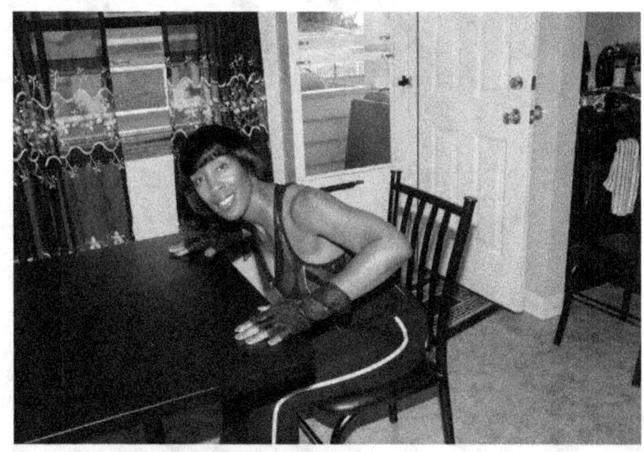

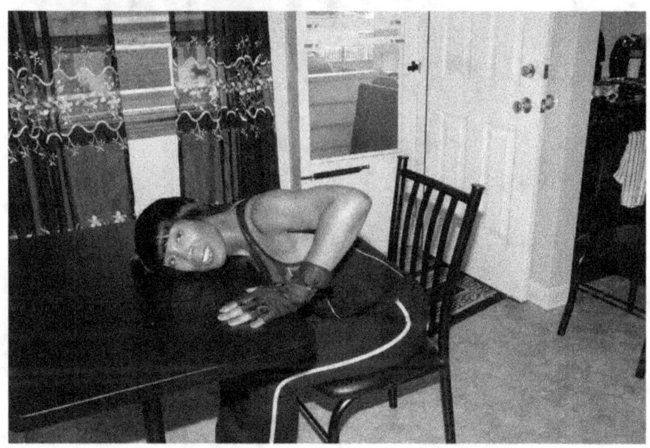

Wall Push-Up

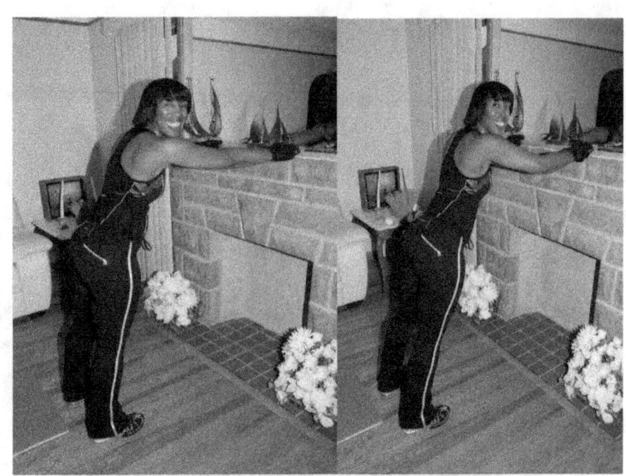

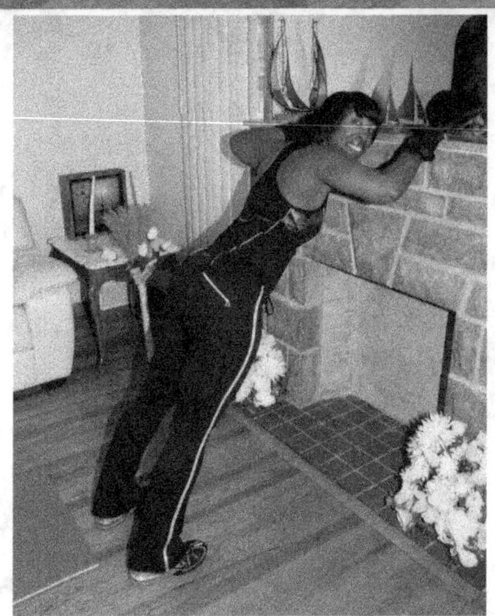

Floor Push-Up

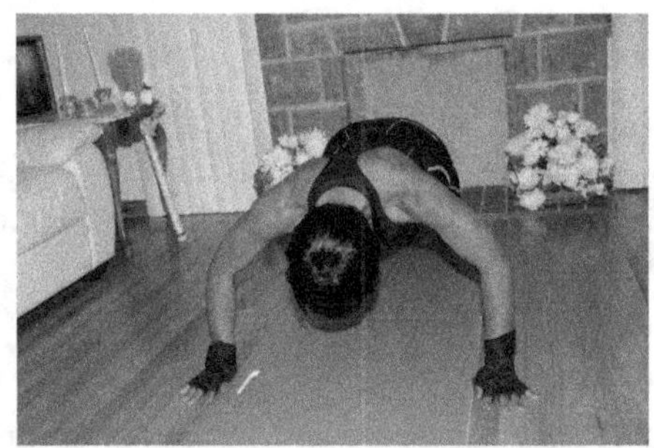

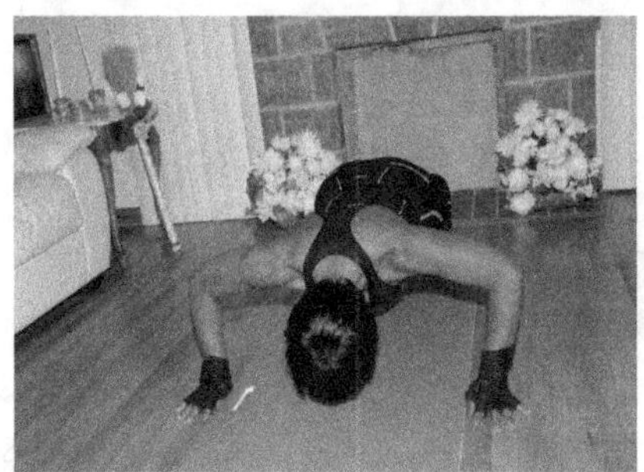

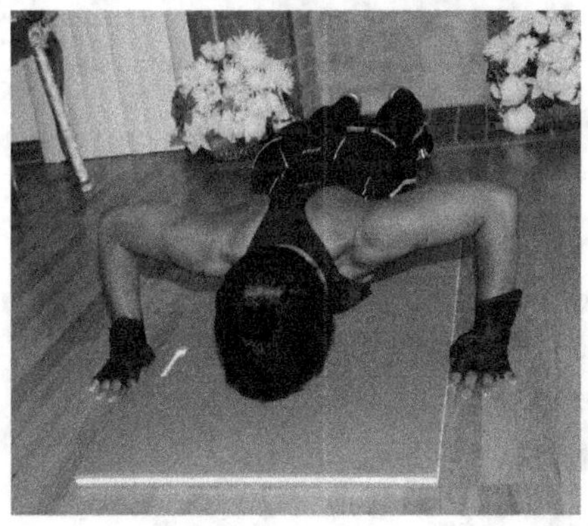

Family Ab-Work

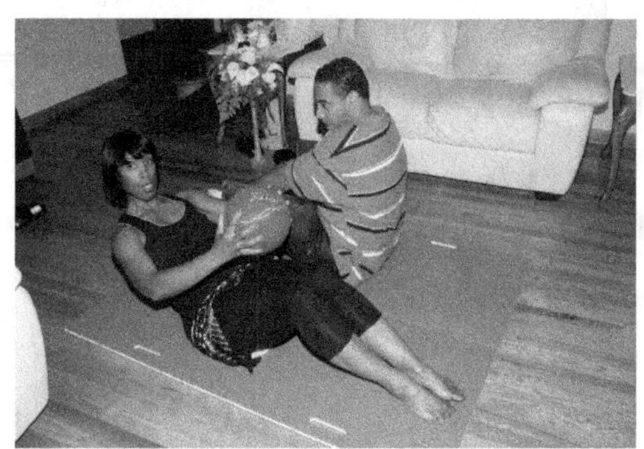

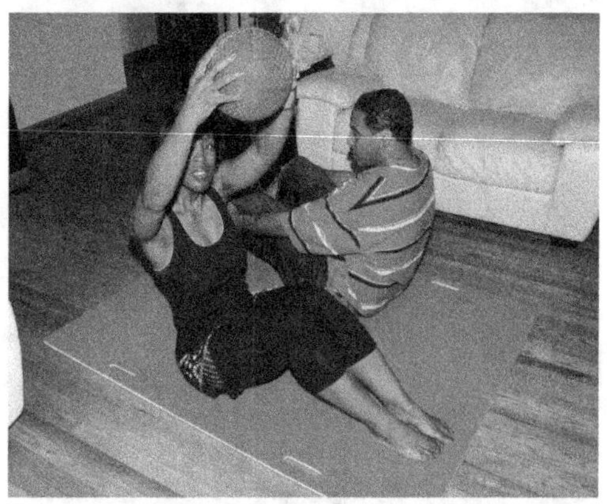

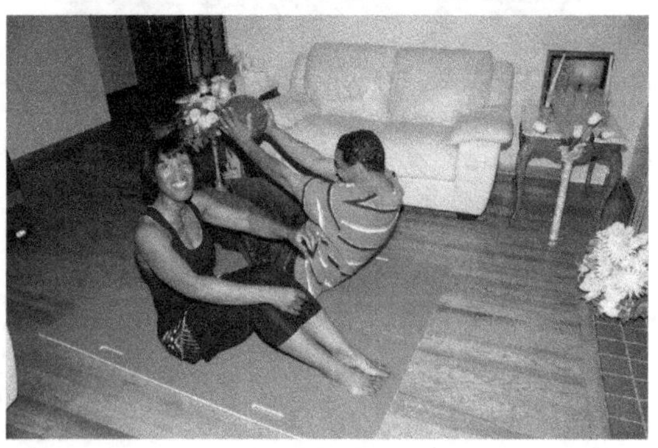

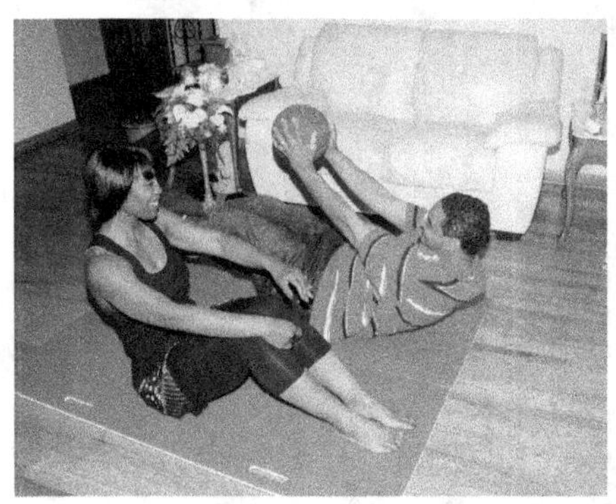

Yoga Poses

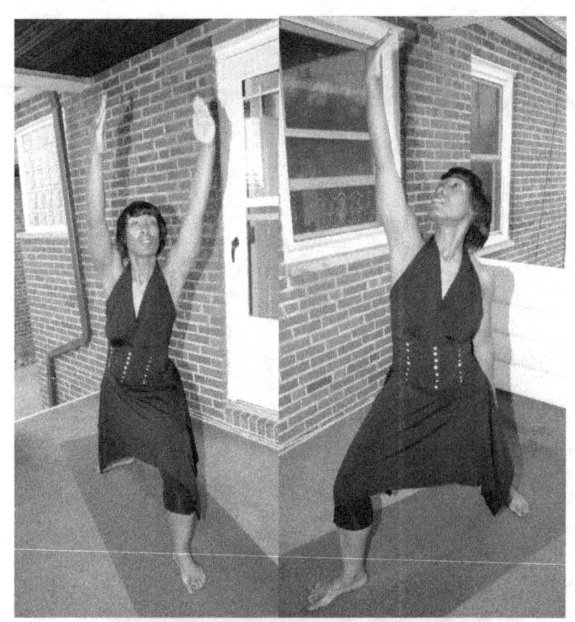

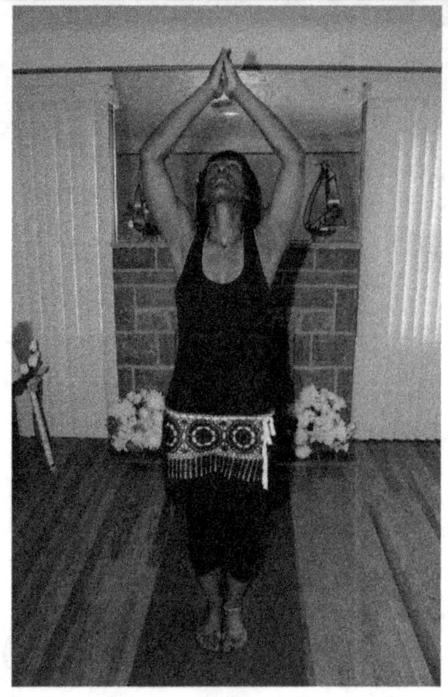

Family Fun

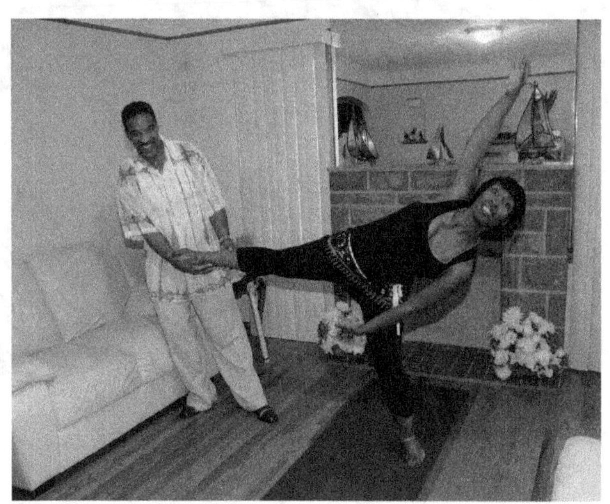

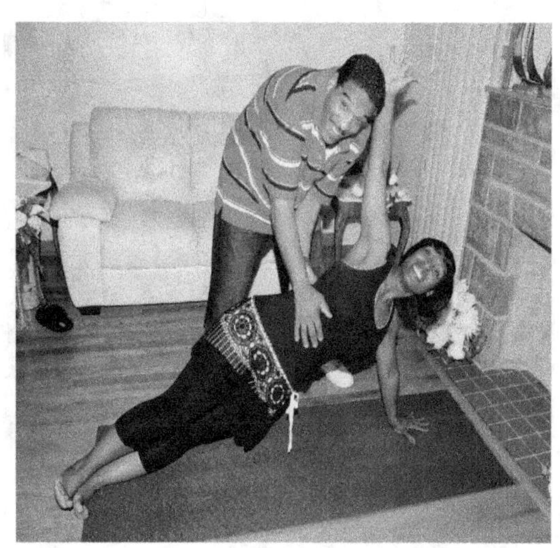

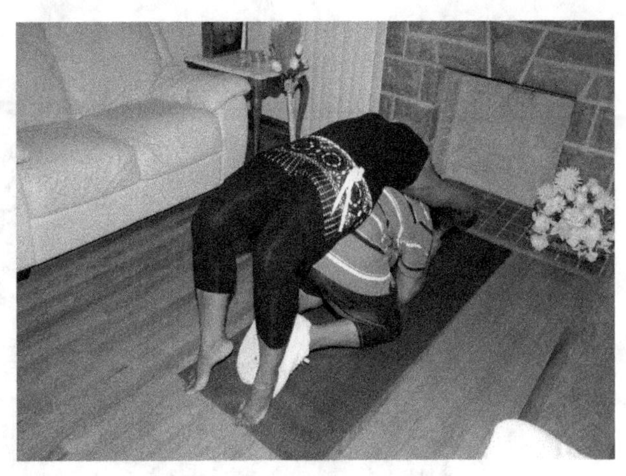

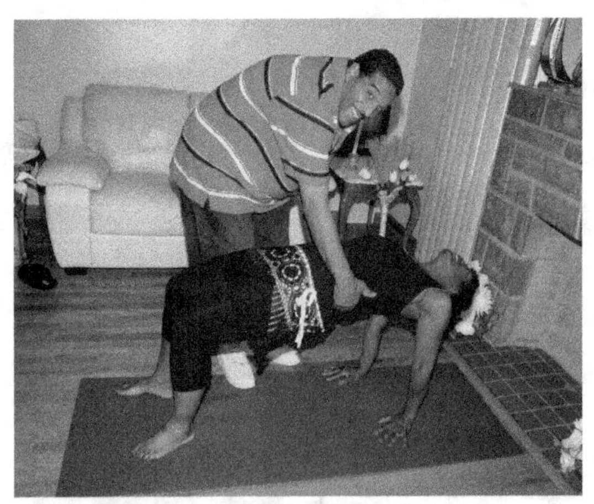

ABOUT THE AUTHOR

Through God's grace, mercy, and guidance, Dr. Fredina Usher-Weems is a Health and Fitness Specialist, Manager, and Consultant, which includes the following fitness areas:

1. Group Fitness Seminar
2. Health and Fitness Motivational Speaker
3. Toddler/Children Youth Fitness Seminar
4. Teen Health and Fitness Trainer Seminar
5. Senior Citizen Health and Fitness Trainer Seminar
6. Martial Artist Trainer/Instructor/Seminar

Fredi is known for her image as a "Fitness Motivator." People attend the fitness sessions suffering from depression, low self-esteem, discouragement, and hopelessness. After several sessions, participants develop a better self-image and increased self-respect, became physically fit, and develop/maintain a healthy outlook on daily living.

Training offered through Fredina Usher-Weems is special because it appeals to a variety of individual at different fitness levels, such as children, teenagers, senior citizens, athletes, weight loss individuals, martial artists, blue collar workers, entrepreneurs, corporations, homemakers, and bariatric patients.

Fredina Usher-Weems has a passion for the field of health and wellness. Her journey began at the young age of twelve when neighborhood friends and family members declared her the fitness instructor at the daycare center her parents owned in Cleveland, Ohio. When the kids came in, they started their morning off doing laps, jumping jacks, and push-ups.

She has a double major degree in Business Administration and in Health and Fitness. She also has a Master's degree in Art and Religion along with a Master of Divinity in Professionalism. She has a Wellness, Doctorate in Ministry from Ashland Theological Seminary. Her final ascent in education will be receiving a Master of Arts in Pastoral Counseling and Leadership.

While pursuing double majors in undergraduate studies, she taught aerobics classes, and gave health and fitness presentations at Cleveland area fitness centers. She also provided services to Girl Scout events, Cleveland Clinic's fitness facilities, Health Expression and the Cleveland Public School System. She holds several certifications including the American College of Sports Medicine, the Aerobic Fitness Association of America, and the Cooper Institute in Dallas, TX.

She currently carries the distinction of Distinguished Presenter in public speaking from Toastmasters International. She has been seen on local TV, written for Cleveland Clinic's Today's Daily Dose, The Health Hub Blog, and has contributed to the YouBeauty web site, The List (Channel Five) and other national publications.

Through her travels and thirty years of experience, she has developed a mantra: "Getting fit is about learning to love, respect, and appreciate you. Sometimes you fall, and that's ok!" Now, as a licensed Pastor/Minister, she is determined to maintain a healthy lifestyle, preach the Gospel through fitness, and educate and train others how to live a life of wellness based on biblical principles.

Her love and desire to worship and serve God by living a healthy lifestyle has motivated Fredi to guide others down the fitness road. God desires that mankind worship and serve him physically with a physically fit body, mind, and soul. Therefore, she witnesses, "with God as my pilot, determination, education and prayer, I will provide you, the reader, with a roadmap to keep you on a successful health and fitness journey."

Enjoy!
Have a blessed work-out.

Fredi

Dr. Usher-Weems can be reached at:

wonderfullymade 497@att.net and

fredina@wonderfullymadeinc.com

website www.wonderfullymadeinc.com

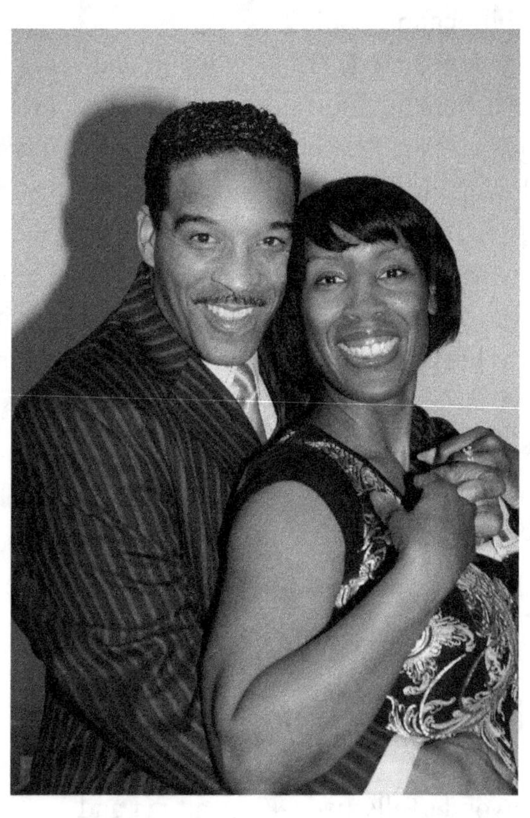